THE SILENT INTRUDER

A personal journey
of living with cancer

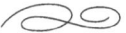

JAN WILLS-COLLINS

The Silent Intruder
Copyright © Jan Wills-Collins 2025

Disclaimer

This book details the author's personal experiences with and opinions about cancer. The author is not a healthcare provider.

The content of this book is not intended to be used to diagnose, treat, cure or prevent any condition or disease. Please consult with your own physician or healthcare specialist regarding the suggestions and recommendations made in this book.

The content is based on the author's knowledge and experience in the field of cancer treatment and does not provide a comprehensive coverage of all the treatment options available to cancer patients. Readers are advised to consult with a qualified healthcare professional before beginning any traditional or alternative treatment program.

The author and publisher disclaim any liability for injuries, accidents or adverse health outcomes that may result from the information provided in this book. Always listen to your body, respect your limitations and seek professional guidance if you have any concerns or questions.

All rights reserved. This book may not be reproduced in whole or part, stored, posted on the internet, or transmitted in any form or by any means, electronic or mechanical, or by photocopying, recording, sharing or other means, without written permission from the author of this book. All content found online or offline without written permission is in breach of copyright law and, therefore, renders you liable for damages and at risk of prosecution.

Cover art titled *Gratitude* by Robin Ranga. Used with permission.

Published by Jan Wills-Collins with assistance from
Ignite & Write Publishing www.igniteandwritepublishing.com

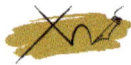

ISBN: 978-0-646-71869-9 (paperback)

Dedication

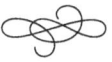

I have written this book with love and a deep understanding for all my friends and loved ones who have travelled this same road.

Some have lost their battle; some of us are still fighting.

Forever in my thoughts are my brother John, my parents Ron and Noeline Butt, my children's father Ross Wills, grandparents Rose and Doug Wills, as well as Dennis, Mary, Joe, Monty, Terry, Faye, Nita and Reg – all members of my cancer support group – who all succumbed to 'the crab'.

I dedicate this book to all those who have walked the cancer journey and to doctors Rick and Fleur, whose guidance and swift action with my initial referrals helped me navigate this frightening path.

A heartfelt thank you to Robin Ranga for her inspirational cover, *Gratitude* – a perfect reflection of the love and support that sustain those of us still on this road.

Contents

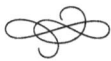

Introduction	1
The first visit	3
First thoughts	7
In the beginning	13
Bladder cancer explained	17
A journey of healing	21
Helpful therapies	25
Post-infusion	27
Roadblocks to recovery	33
Redefining normal	37
Using humour to cope	39
Communicating with other sufferers	41
Reflection	47
Resources	49
About the author	51
References	53

Introduction

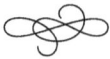

Why am I writing this book? To be honest, I'm not entirely sure. What I do know is that I hope my voice and my thoughts might, in some small way, resonate with and help others on their cancer journey.

This is not my first book. In 2020, I published *Hidden Scars of Polio*, in which I wrote about my experience with this terrible virus. Prior to the 1955 introduction of the vaccine, polio was a major cause of disability in children. I was aged eleven, my sister only aged two, when we were diagnosed in the midst of the polio global pandemic of 1952. It was a traumatic experience. My sister slipped into a coma, while I was momentarily paralysed down the right side of my body. When she roused from the coma, my sister was able to go home to be cared for by my parents, but I was to remain in the hospital for many months. My life changed dramatically, with years of ongoing problems that I managed to overcome.

Thankfully, I was able to go on to lead a happy, active life. Polio had been my biggest challenge, but I made it through. And now, I find myself back in a similar situation. This time aged eighty-four and facing another frightening threat to my life.

Numb best describes my feelings when I was first hit with the realisation that I had yet another hurdle to navigate. Of course, a cancer diagnosis brings many different emotions with it.

Those thoughts: *It isn't fair. How is this really happening? Why do I have to endure more pain and anguish in this lifetime?*

They circled my mind on many an occasion.

Polio had been replaced by that dreaded 'c' word – cancer. It was infiltrating my world and my family's world. Like with polio, cancer also carried stigmas. Your friends are either supportive, over supportive or simply too afraid to see you.

And believe this if you will, some of those people in my life even thought it could be contagious.

It was just before Christmas 2022 when I received my bladder cancer diagnosis. I made the decision to get on with my life – to fight – and this is where my story begins.

The first visit

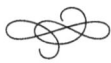

The only sound I could hear was the 'hmmm' being made by the doctor who was doing my ultrasound.

He might not have been the most communicative of medical professionals, but I trusted his diagnostic skills implicitly.

I could feel and hear my heart beating faster and louder as I tentatively asked, 'So, you can see something?'

Surely that was what his monosyllable murmur had meant.

With the doctor wearing his mask, I was unable to read his expression.

'Possibly,' was all he offered.

I persisted. 'Is it a tumour?'

Again, very brief dialogue.

'Probably.'

He continued after a brief pause: 'Who referred you to me?'

'Doctor Fleur,' I replied.

So, I went back to my referring doctor. Dr Fleur was working at our local Whangamatā Medical Centre as a locum seconded from Holland. And what a blessing she was, so caring and attentive to patient needs.

What followed was a whirlwind of referrals as she quickly organised further ultrasounds and specialist appointments.

As I stood at the reception counter organising the slew of appointments, unbeknownst to me, my husband, Richard, walked into the medical centre. He saw me there with Dr Fleur's arm around me. He was panicked into thinking I was going to die. He turned and went back to the car with a rush of thoughts going through his mind.

Minutes later, when I went out to the car with no knowledge that he was already in a downhill spiral, I burst out with a 'it's not good'.

Already thinking the worst, he stared at me in disbelief, as if I had said something so blatanly obvious. Then and there, we decided to get on with the task at hand.

Was this even real? How could this be happening?

'It will be okay,' we reassured each other. 'Let's get this show on the road and onto the path of recovery.'

Dr Fleur was so valuable in organising my diagnostic appointments. Quite conveniently, it so happened, I was privately booked to go to Takapuna for a mammogram. Takapuna, which is located on the North Shore of Auckland, is a two-and-a-half-hour drive from our hometown. The clinic there very obligingly organised an ultrasound of my bladder that same day. This procedure confirmed the initial diagnosis of a bladder tumour.

An urgent visit to the urologist was the next step. Dr Fleur once again was so helpful, and we were able to secure an appointment for the next day. It was to be with Dr Leyland, a urology specialist from Waikato.

This appointment was actually conducted in Dr Leyland's clinic situated in Morrinsville, a relatively short one-and-a-half-hour drive for us. I have nothing but praise for this man. So gentle and understanding, he put my husband and me completely at ease, even as I faced fears about what lay ahead.

THE FIRST VISIT

This visit again confirmed the presence of a tumour and the urgency for surgery. I guess 'lucky' is a strange word to use in the circumstances, but lucky I was.

As the head of urology at Waikato Hospital, Dr Leyland arranged for me to be on the operating list the following Monday – only two days after seeing him. My husband and I were so grateful to have so little time to fret and worry.

So, from the time of diagnosis to surgery, it was barely a week.

First thoughts

Without warning, suddenly your world is turned upside down. Life has a way of blindsiding you with the unexpected.

For me, that moment arrived when I heard the word 'cancer', and even more threatening, the words 'bladder cancer' for the first time.

'Not me,' I say to myself. 'I'm the carer – the person who worries about everyone else.'

Life had thrown me a curveball. My mind was racing and my brain was in overdrive.

You can't do this to me.

My parents both had cancer; my brother had his life cut short at 38 years from this dreaded disease.

My sister is in remission from breast cancer. My two sons lost their dad to cancer.

I have been blessed with a wonderful husband, second time around, and we still have plans for things to do together.

I want to see my beautiful 17-year-old granddaughter mature and settle into her chosen career.

I have to see our three-year-old twin grandchildren – our beautiful miracle babies – off to school.

Dear God, I want my children and grandchildren to remember me with as much love as I have for them.

Fight or flight – I have to fight.

Why is it that we talk about 'our cancer journey' as though it is the main star of the show? Truly, our life is the real journey. It can be easy to forget that when you are handed such a cruel sentence.

When bladder cancer enters your life, it is not just a fleeting guest. No, it becomes your constant companion.

And it isn't a solitary journey. It follows a path that ripples through relationships, family and friends.

The question my mind posed bore down on my soul: *How do I navigate this? How do I continue to maintain my connections while dealing with my treatment?*

These moments were the beginning of a journey that reshaped my life, not only physically, but emotionally as well. I learnt quickly that open communication is essential – in good times and the bad.

The moment the news of my diagnosis spread, it became real. For sure, it was heartening to know that I was surrounded by so much care and love, but sometimes, that too feels overwhelming.

A cancer diagnosis creates an influx of inquiries – a deluge of calls and messages flow in. The daily phone calls from well-meaning friends were, of course, coming from their desire to support me. Sometimes, though, they added to my stress; a constant reminder of the intruder I was now harbouring within.

'Let me know if there's anything I can do.' I heard it plenty. My suggestion? Don't call – just do it. While at the supermarket, phone your friend, ask if they need you to pick something up. Trust me, it is appreciated.

There was also the: 'You have cancer, you look so well' comments. While that is a good thing, sometimes the person going through the illness feels differently, and although they may look well, perhaps their mental state is not in a healthy place.

And the hardest one to swallow that was thrown at me: 'I know what you are going through'.

Really and truly, no one knows. We all experience our situation in our own way. Perhaps, try saying something simple like, 'This must be so hard for you'.

Dealing with inquiries isn't only about managing your own responses, but it is also about helping others understand your boundaries. Naturally, people want to show their support, and it comes from a place of love and empathy.

So, although I wanted to manage the diagnoses in my own way, I knew I had to respect the connection needed by all of those close to me.

It was very heartwarming to know and feel many cared, but this journey was mine – it still is – and only I knew and understood how I needed to handle it. I needed to take ownership, and in doing so, it created a challenge in balancing my desires with those around me.

Understanding came more naturally from my family and friends when they realised and accepted how I wanted to play the game. I continued to attend my various group meetings and kept myself busy with my garden club secretarial duties.

Crying and stressing did not help me, or those around me, but rest assured, there were some dark days. Cancer brings with it a deep uncertainty.

What I have learnt is that cancer does not hold back and neither should we. Set your boundaries – you will need them.

My inspirations that kept and continue to keep me sane.

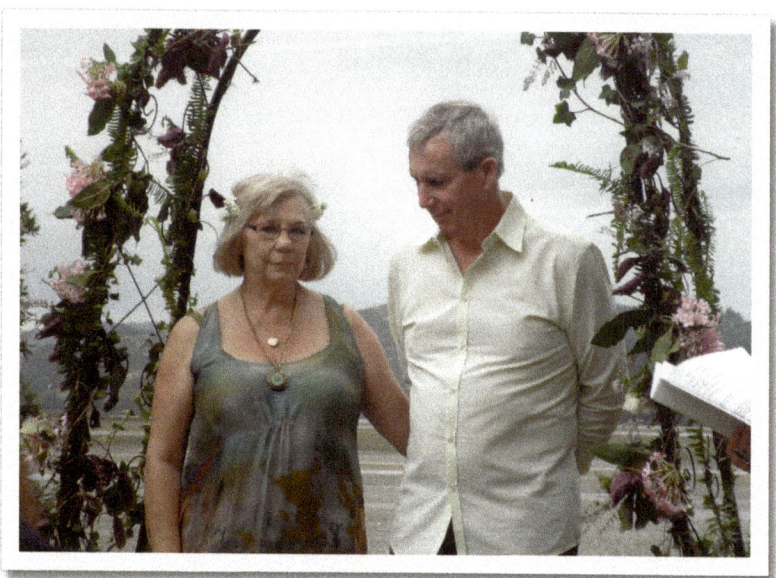

Richard and I, 2012.

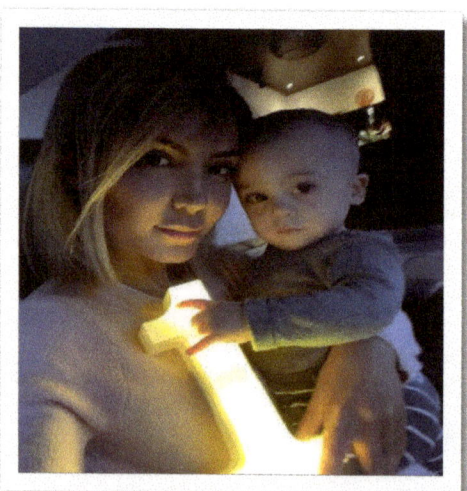
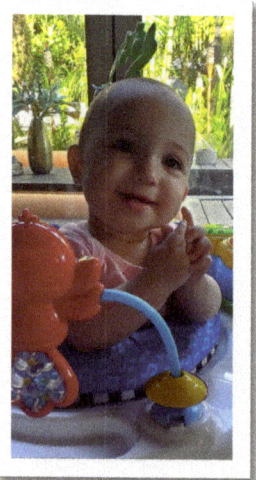

Our twins, Zac and Zara, with their beautiful mum Mona.

FIRST THOUGHTS

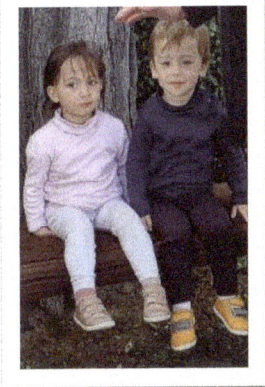 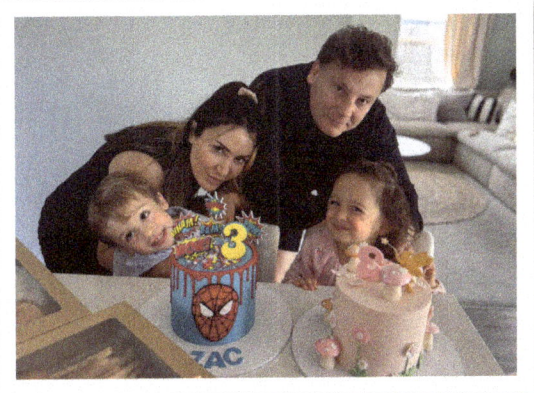

The twins, pictured with Guy and Mona, turn three.

My beautiful granddaughter Billie, pictured with me. 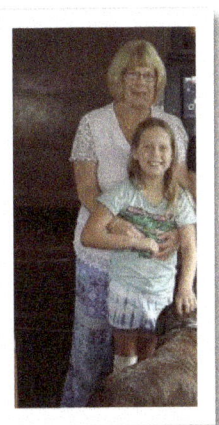 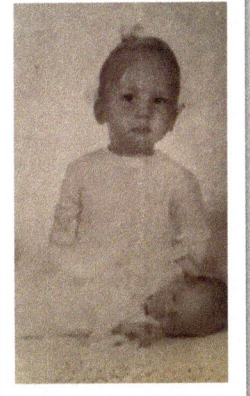 My two special boys, my sons.

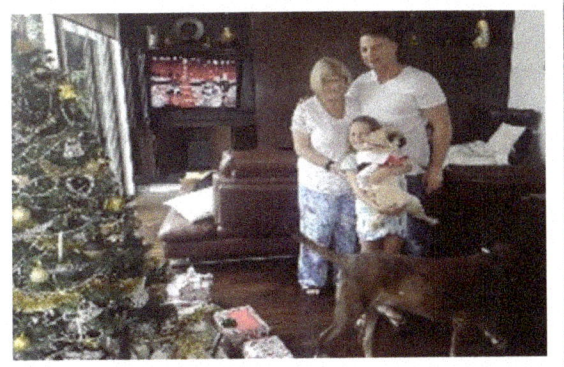 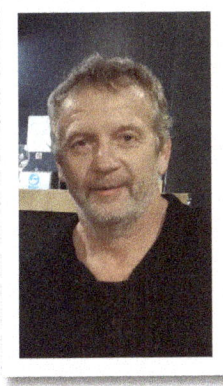

Me with Guy, my eldest, and Billie, my granddaughter.   My youngest, Scott.

In the beginning

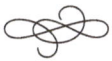

I had been happily enjoying a trip away with my garden club, visiting some amazing spots in and around Cambridge, a town in Waikato, New Zealand, when I suddenly felt terribly ill and began haemorrhaging from the bladder.

The horror of seeing a toilet bowl full of blood and large clots was absolutely terrifying. I was sick to my stomach, and truthfully, very frightened. With only two more days left of the trip, I decided to wait it out. Looking back now, those last few days are hazy. I had fallen into a daze.

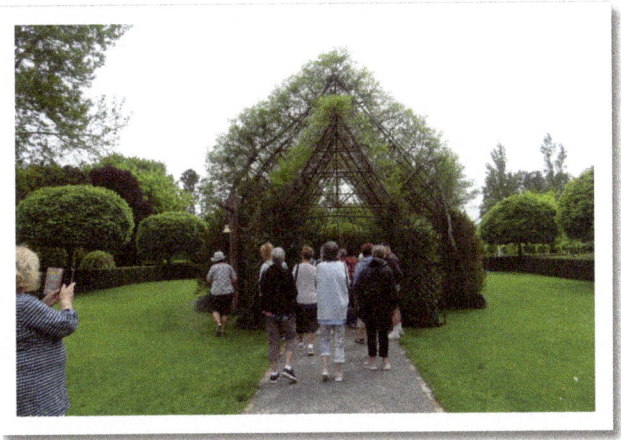

The beautiful Tree Church in Cambridge, Waikato, New Zealand.

I was awake most of those nights imagining every scenario these symptoms could be caused by, or what they might develop into. I must admit though, not once did I actually consider I could have cancer – surely that couldn't happen to me.

Once I returned home, I went straight to the doctor where there was some hope, with the initial thought being that it was just an infection. Antibiotics did nothing; the bleeding continued and, looking back, I realise the signs were there.

I certainly didn't connect it with previous bleeding I had noticed, thinking it was just an 'ageing issue'. I recalled how some time back, my daughter-in-law had been concerned upon finding blood in the toilet. I was quick to deny any knowledge of it when my son spoke to me about it.

It was very close to Christmas time, with post-COVID restrictions still in place in some areas, especially the medical environment. I am forever grateful to doctors Fleur and Rick Budenseik, who was also a locum at the Whangamatā Medical Centre, for their care and for being instrumental in getting me referrals so quickly. The constant phone calls from both these doctors gave me reassurance that they cared, and hope that this problem was being addressed.

As you have already read, my visits to the medical centre led to the ultrasounds, which were then followed by a visit to the urology specialist, who confirmed the presence of this tumour.

Dr John Leyland was wonderful – so gentle and understanding.

Picture this, if you will. You are in the doctor's office, and you hear the words: 'I'm afraid you have a tumour. You have bladder cancer and we need to organise surgery to remove the tumour. It is reasonably urgent.'

Reasonably urgent? *That can't be good.*

The initial shock of hearing the words 'cancer' and 'tumour' said out loud was surreal. Then the reality began to surface and my mind, once again, went into overdrive.

IN THE BEGINNING

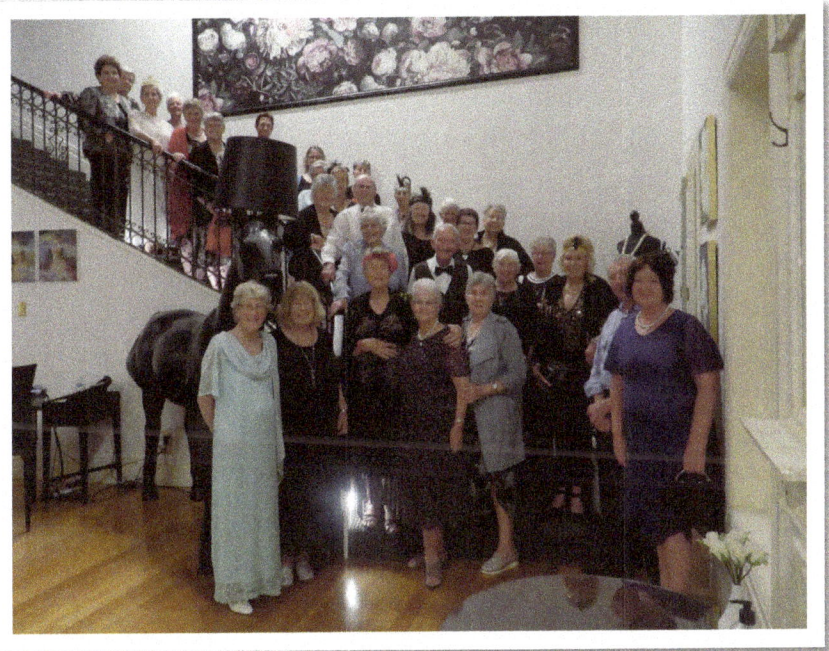

Garden club trip 2022, The Henley Hotel Cambridge.

Cancer! I have bladder cancer!

A rush of emotions – fear, disbelief, anger – all surfaced within me. When you are told that you have cancer, your emotions ebb and flow like the sea.

In that instant, I embarked on a path I never imagined, a path that demanded strength I never knew I had.

Cancer! How do I tell my family?

A diagnosis of chronic illness intrudes unexpectedly into the lives of many close to you. My children had already suffered from watching their father succumb to cancer. I did not want to subject them to any extra pain or stress.

Let's play this down and just get on with whatever I have to do to expel this unwanted guest from my body.

Bladder cancer changes your life in ways you never anticipated, and the shift in perspective that occurs during your journey is unfathomable. It has changed my life, but not who I am.

Cancer knows no boundaries and affects people from all walks of life.

As the diagnosis settled in, the whirlwind of treatment discussions began, with the surgery emerging as my immediate option.

Medical jargon, treatment options and survival rates became part of my personal vocabulary.

It was of utmost importance that my husband was included in discussions and my family kept informed, as they were part of my journey.

Bladder cancer explained

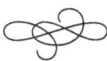

So, how exactly does bladder cancer form, and what does it do to the body?

According to the Cancer Council, a person's cells normally grow and multiply in an orderly way. However, damaged genes can cause them to behave abnormally, and this is when they can grow into a lump called a tumour. Tumours can be benign (not cancerous) or malignant (cancerous).[1]

Your bladder

The bladder is a hollow, stretchy organ in the lower part of your abdomen that stores urine before it leaves your body through your urethra.

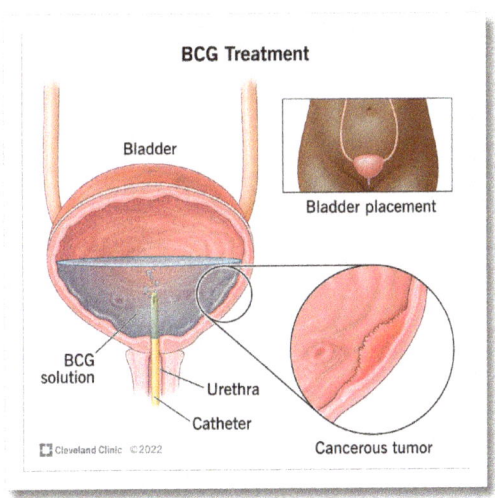

The Cleveland Clinic's diagram for Bacillus Calmette-Guérin (BCG) treatment.[2]

The following information is specific to bladder cancer only.

Occurrence of bladder cancer is three times higher in men than among women. Moreover, women are generally diagnosed with a more severe tumour stage and have a poorer prognosis.[3]

Bladder cancer can occur in several forms. Urothelial carcinoma, previously known as transitional cell carcinoma, is the most common type, accounting for eighty to ninety per cent of cases. It begins in the urothelial cells that line the innermost layer of the bladder wall. Squamous cell carcinoma, which represents about one to two per cent of cases, develops in the thin, flat cells that form the lining of the bladder. A much rarer form, adenocarcinoma, makes up around one per cent of cases and arises from mucus-producing cells in the bladder. This type is generally considered to be invasive.[4]

Signs and symptoms may include blood in the urine, painful/frequent urination, pelvic pain and back pain.[5]

How is it treated?

As detailed on the Cancer Council's website, bladder cancer can be treated in several ways, depending on how advanced the disease is. One common approach is surgery, specifically a procedure called transurethral resection of bladder tumour (TURBT). This involves the use of a cystoscope fitted with a wire loop, which the doctor uses to remove any tumours. In some cases, the base of the tumour may be burned, or high-energy lasers may be used to damage or destroy the cancer cells.

Immunotherapy is another option for non-invasive bladder cancers. This can involve the use of a vaccine called Bacillus Calmette-Guérin (BCG), originally developed to prevent tuberculosis. BCG helps stimulate the immune system to attack cancer cells and may help stop or delay the progression of bladder cancer.

Chemotherapy is also used to target and destroy cancer cells. In cases of non-invasive bladder cancer, chemotherapy drugs can be delivered directly into the bladder – a method known as intravesical chemotherapy. For more advanced, invasive bladder cancers, surgery is the most common treatment. However, radiation therapy (radiotherapy) is sometimes used as an alternative, and in certain situations, chemotherapy may be added to the treatment plan.[6]

More about BCG

Unlike oral or injectable drugs, BCG targets cancer cells inside your bladder without having a negative impact on the rest of your body. Before beginning BCG treatment, local anaesthesia is given to numb the area and keep you comfortable. Next, a catheter is placed into the urethra and the BCG solution is injected into the bladder. The BCG solution needs to come in contact with the cancer cells to kill them.[7]

The schedule

The initial BCG cancer treatment occurs weekly for six weeks. If the treatment is working, a patient may then be given BCG weekly for three weeks at the three-, six-, and twelve-month marks. This may be continued for up to three years.[7]

Advantages of BCG

When performed in combination with TURBT, BCG treatment is the most effective treatment for high-risk non-invasive bladder cancer. This includes those that have not invaded the bladder wall muscle. According to information from the Cleveland Clinic, BCG cancer treatment can slow tumour growth and reduce the need for a cystectomy.[7]

A journey of healing

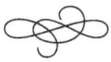

My clinical information stated, 'Patient presenting for an elective transurethral resection of bladder tumour'.

The tumour was described as a 'large three-centimetre tumour on a narrow stalk-left lateral wall'.

As an older person – young at heart but 84 chronologically – my mind was racing about the what-ifs. I could not sleep very well as I started to worry about the anaesthetic and the surgery.

Can I come through this?

Having had polio at eleven years of age and now being subjected to post-polio complications, my lungs are compromised. So, I was worried about the surgery.

There was no need and I give my utmost praise to everyone involved in my care at the Waikato Hospital and the preparation I received from the entire medical team. No stone was left unturned in my pre-surgery checks, explanations of procedures and post-surgery care.

The size and degree of invasion were paramount in the decision for my treatment.

The tumour was removed by a transurethral resection with no complications during or post-surgery. I awoke to find a three-way catheter had been inserted in theatre and I was on continuous bladder irrigations.

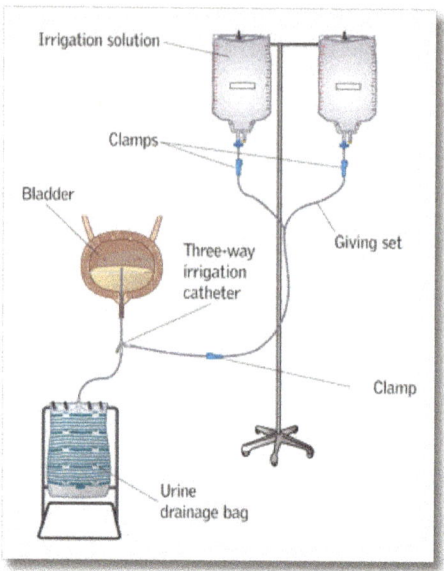

The three-way catheter as explained by expert nurse Beverly Cutts on rcni.com.[8]

This is the post-surgery management normally used following urological surgery. It is a procedure that flushes the bladder with a sterile liquid. It also removes urine from the body at the same time. An operation on your urinary system can cause blood clots and debris, which in turn, can cause blockage and subsequent infection. The three-way catheter allows fluid to flow in and out of the bladder simultaneously, allowing for full drainage.

The first post-surgery visit to the urologist was another hurdle I had to overcome. I was informed the tumour had come back from histology as being aggressive.

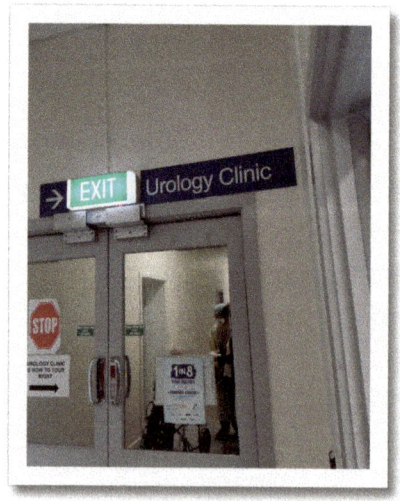

Waikato Hospital.

And so began my BCG treatment – an experience that would have been far less tolerable if it wasn't for my wonderful nurse, Maureen. With her compassionate nature, understanding and gentleness, Maureen made my weekly Friday infusions at the Thames Hospital a more comfortable experience.

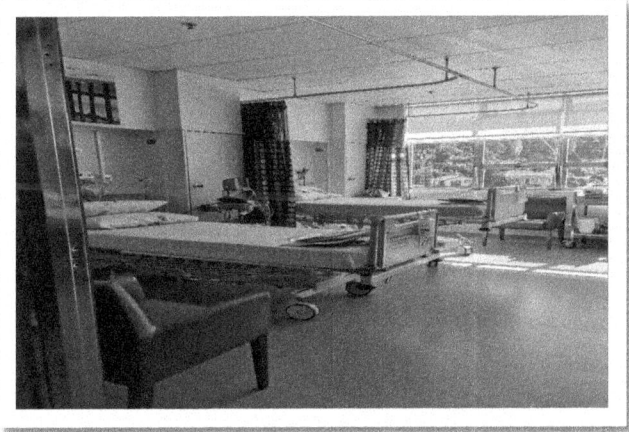

My second home, Thames Hospital, level three, where I had my infusions.

There were, of course, trials and tribulations stemming from my initial visits. I'm not sure if it was my anatomy or plain nervousness, but my first visits were fraught with much difficulty for Maureen to administer the infusion into the right place.

I asked Maureen if a male or female infusion was easier. Without hesitation she replied, 'A man of course, as there is only one way to navigate.'

I'm happy to say that after those difficulties were overcome, Friday infusions were never a problem again.

The waiting room

Every waiting room has its own atmosphere. For patients awaiting results, or already coping with a cancer diagnosis, we don't want to be reminded of why we are there – we need something to make us smile. For me, I found the waiting room at Thames Hospital full of humour, which can help during those moments. It became a place where I could actually make and nurture new friendships. It was a time of sharing and listening to each other, even with our modesty sometimes compromised.

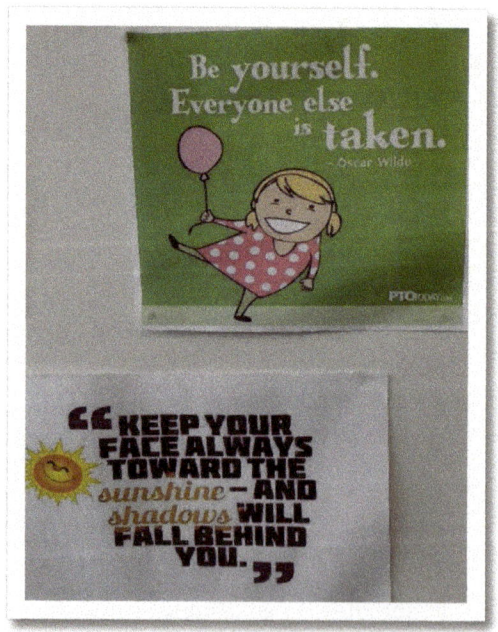

Some inspiring posters in the waiting room at the Waikato hospital.

Helpful therapies

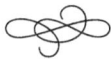

It is my belief that, alongside conventional treatment, it is okay to enter into other helpful therapies. Realise of course, I am not advocating or promoting alternative therapies. A patient must never stop tried and true conventional treatments.

In my case, the therapies I pursued were purely for pain relief and stress management. Fortunately, I did find some of these treatments – and the wonderful people delivering them – beneficial in navigating the journey.

You really don't need to be battling cancer or any other life-threatening situation to visit these wonderful people. Sometimes our everyday lives need a boost, so don't be afraid to reach out.

I found acupuncture a helpful tool to address pain, and was lucky enough to find Katrina who had studied in China at a hospital that specialised in oncology. Katrina was a breath of fresh air and so knowledgeable. To this day, I look forward to my session with her and always come away with renewed strength to face another day.

Another support mechanism I was fortunate enough to partake in was a process called 'havening'. During my working life, I taught and practised peer support and critical incident stress management, so I was no stranger to counselling and this type of process. My sessions were with Penny, whose compassion and kindness were second to none.

Havening is a technique that mainly involves visualisation. It is a psychosensory therapy that uses touch, eye movements and other sensory inputs to address anxiety, trauma and other emotional issues by training the brain to respond differently to stressful situations.

During my working life as a health and safety manager in the New Zealand Fire Service, I was heavily involved in trauma management. This meant that I had an understanding of this type of therapy and wasn't afraid to participate.

While there is no scientific evidence supporting its alleged effectiveness, I found it calming and helpful in resolving issues and anxiety, especially at the time when things changed within my cancer support group and some people, those who I believed were my friends, rejected me.

Nutrition was another allied health service that I leaned on. I found Michelle, a must-see guru of nutrition, who shared her in-depth knowledge with me. She reminded me that eating well is an important part of self-care, as a healthy lifestyle can improve energy levels.

Self-care along your cancer journey isn't just driven solely by the medical aspects. It is also important to nurture all your body's needs.

Post-infusion

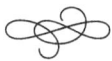

Because my tumour was shown to be aggressive, my time dealing with this cancer would not be over for many months, if ever.

As a deterrent to any future cancer cells that might develop in my bladder, the BCG infusions were to become a regular item in my diary. With the infusion for bladder cancer being given directly into the bladder via a catheter, it was with much apprehension that I presented at the Thames Hospital for the first session.

The procedure was invasive and could be quite humiliating. However, the professionalism and approach from the nurses allayed my fears and every visit after that initial one was not a problem.

Post-infusion can be a different story and challenging to navigate. Firstly, you are not allowed to go to the toilet for two hours after the infusion. So, that one-hour drive home could be uncomfortable for me. The other issue is that you are unable to use any public restroom due to the infusion containing a live tuberculosis vaccine. The infusion solution can be lethal if it contaminates you or another person.

Once home, I had to use a separate toilet (I do not know what people do when they only have one!) and then soak the bowl in bleach for fifteen minutes afterwards. A real nuisance all round, but a necessary evil when dealing with this type of infusion.

This may seem a trivial concern, but when you are in a state of stress, these are the little things that really agitate and upset you. I am told that some people fly through the infusions with no problems, but for me, it was miserable, and I had pain for several days after each infusion. This was followed by a few comfortable days until the next visit. Some treatments left me with flu-like symptoms.

But let's be grateful. I am not losing my hair, and I am not fading away.

I dreaded those weekly Fridays for another reason – the journey to Thames itself. In recent years, I had become somewhat of a nervous passenger, and navigating the winding hills and steep drops was not pleasant in my already fraught state of mind.

To add to my stress and fear of travel, in February 2023, a severe, destructive tropical cyclone named Gabrielle devastated parts of the North Island of New Zealand.

Significant damage was caused to State Highway 25a in the Coromandel Peninsula, causing road closures and subsequently cutting off parts of the peninsula.

What did this mean for us?

With no bridge between Whangamatā and Thames, there was no road access through this route. This meant we had to go through Waihi and the Karangahake Gorge every Friday to Thames.

This certainly added to the stress of the day and the worry of getting home in time to go to the toilet, compounded by my aversion to driving through winding hills.

One particular corner in the gorge faces high cliffs and is particularly nasty. So, I became adept at checking my phone in need of a distraction when we approached this stretch of the gorge.

Fortunately, I was able to hold on and make it home to the toilet each time. I got very good at this, and during the time we had to go through the Karangahake Gorge, we were able to stop at a wonderful café for Richard to have some lunch. The Waikino Station Café was a must-stop with its vintage suitcases, lace curtains and an old-fashioned baking set, giving that yesteryear feeling.

With our regular weekly visit, we got to know the staff. I'm not sure why, but one Friday, Richard disclosed to the gentleman who had always served us that I was having treatment for cancer. He explained that I couldn't have coffee just yet, but did love their pies. Well, said gentleman came out from behind the counter, approached our table where I was sitting and gave me a hug and with tears in his eyes, he told me I was very brave. To be honest, I had never thought of my cancer fight as bravery, but I felt heartened that there were caring people like this in the world.

Even so, we didn't get a free pie (I often wonder if that was Richard's motive!).

The road we travelled

Every Friday we set off from our home in Whangamatā, through Waihi and the Karangahake Gorge to get to Thames. Set against a backdrop of native forest, **Whangamatā** is a surf town, located 30 kilometres north of Waihi on the southeast coast of the Coromandel Peninsula in the North Island of New Zealand. It is a stunning four-kilometre-long beach and is a popular holiday destination.

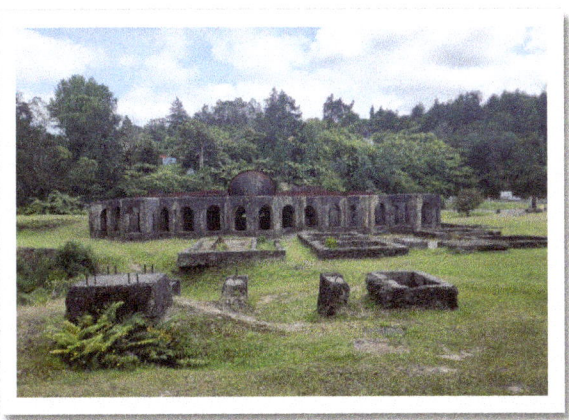

Battery remains along the banks of the Karangahake gorge.

Waihi is a town in the Hauraki District in the North Island of New Zealand. It is known as New Zealand's 'heart of gold' due to its gold mining history spanning three centuries.

Karangahake Gorge is located on State Highway 2 between Paeroa and Waihi, about two hours from Auckland. This heritage site is a labyrinth of tracks and walkways throughout the gorge, with steel and concrete mining relics as reminders of the past.

Thames is the rural centre of the Coromandel, while **Hamilton**, in the Waikato, is the location of the Waikato Hospital.

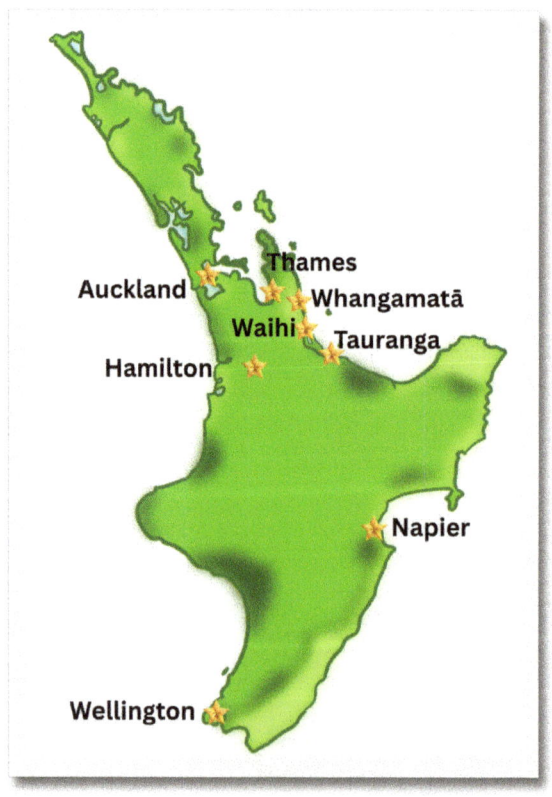

Map of the North Island, New Zealand.
Whangamatā is on the Coromandel Coast.

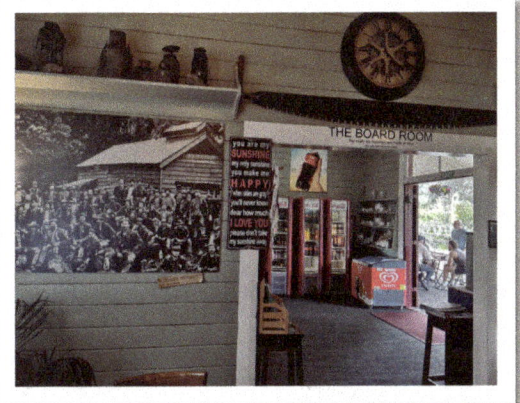 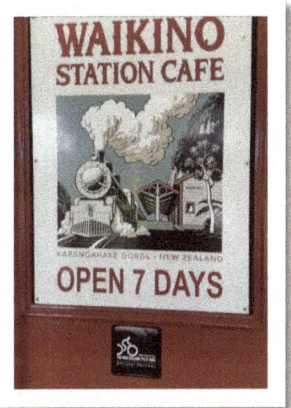

The quaint Waikino Station Café where good memories were made.

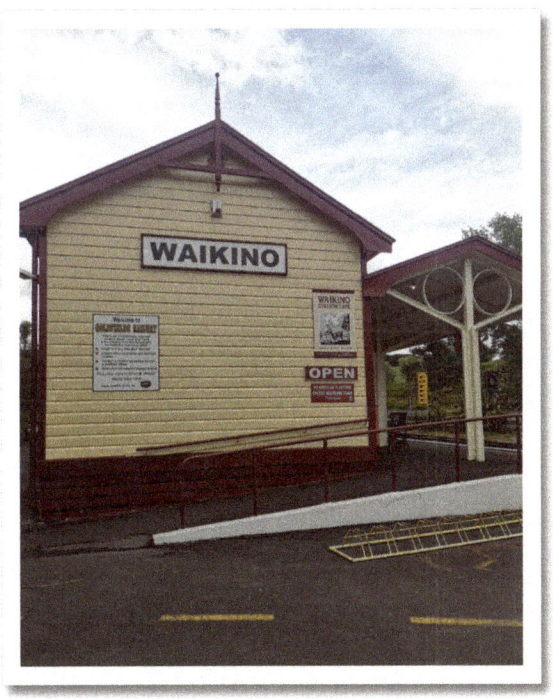

Roadblocks to recovery

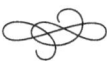

Amidst the trials of treatment, finding a way for normality is vital. One must retain moments of respite from medical appointments and treatments.

My coping mechanism in dealing with this 'thing' hanging over my head was to push it away and not think about it.

Sure, why not pretend it doesn't exist.

With my polio history and current spin-offs from the cancer treatment, I wasn't able to help in the garden, but I could still enjoy gardens and my garden club. Being a part of an organisation where the members were united in their love of flowers and gardens was important to me. As a bonus, I was still able to enjoy their annual trips, which took us to see wonderful gardens and garden art.

Another major player in my coping strategy was the Whangamatā Cancer Support Group of which I was the leader/co-ordinator. I loved this group and all the people in it. My working life as a trained nurse, both in general and mental health, together with my twenty years with the fire service and trauma management, equipped me with counselling skills.

I had been leading the group for more than twelve years, well prior to my own diagnosis. During this time, my training and skills enabled me to listen to people and organise counselling where appropriate. Our group was a happy group of people who really loved getting together each month, and we really enjoyed our monthly meetings.

As a group, we represented all cancer types, and there were no barriers to membership. One just had to be a carer or a cancer sufferer. I often thought the carers suffered more anxiety and stress than the patients themselves so it was a pleasure to welcome them to our group.

We alternated monthly meetings with café visits. Monthly meetings would be just a get-together and chats with maybe the odd quiz and sometimes an appropriate speaker. We were conscious of making these meetings positive and not focusing on why we were together.

Over the years, we organised major fundraising for prostate cancer, breast cancer organisation Sweet Louise and the National Breast Cancer Foundation's Pink Ribbon.

The Pink Ribbon events were outstanding successes, raising more than seven thousand dollars in 2023 and a whopping ten thousand the following year.

These people were a special group, all with a common denominator in their lives. We had either survived cancer, were living with cancer or were closely associated with someone who had suffered from cancer or hadn't survived cancer.

The Whangamatā Cancer Support Christmas event.

So when it was my turn to deal with the cancer intruder, the group became my major support. These people took my mind off the diagnosis – it never seemed real when I was with them. We were a close-knit family.

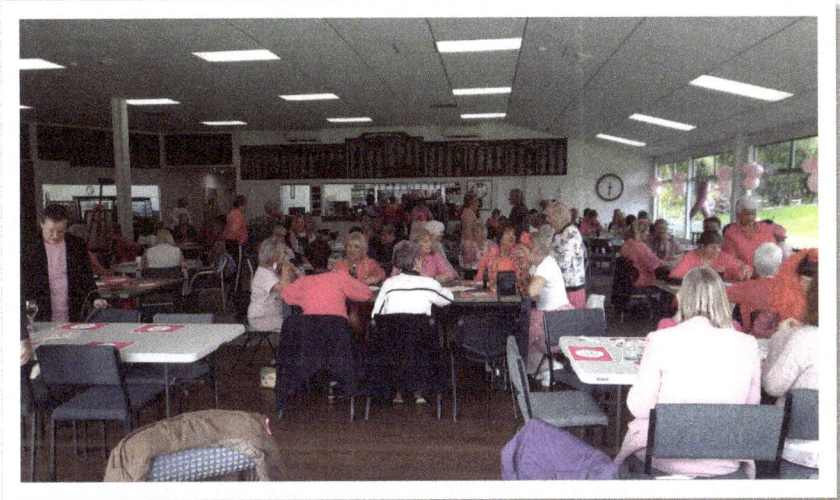

The Pink Ribbon fundraiser luncheon, May 2024.

So, imagine if you can, the shock and hurt that hit me when I was ordered to step down. The National Cancer Society for volunteers ruled that you could not be a volunteer while you had active cancer. There was no warning and the change was to be immediate.

I was gutted, as was my immunotherapy nurse and many friends. This situation could be likened to a critical incident for me. The ripple effect was widespread, and sadly, even caused a rift between some friends.

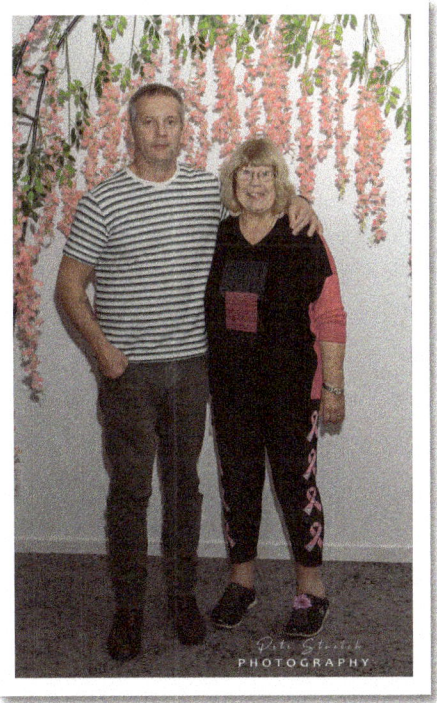

My youngest son, Scott, and me at Pink Ribbon 2024.

I felt bereft and angry that the people involved in this decision-making appeared to have little idea how to walk alongside cancer sufferers, and that what worked for some may not work for others.

I needed companionship and goals to keep me from becoming simply focused on my cancer. I was not able to sit at home and reflect on my cancer. I'm not that person.

Attending the support group was not acceptable at this stage, as I was still very raw from my 'demotion'. So, subsequently, I formed another group, called The Friendship Group, and what a blessing that has been.

I was humbled to see how many people were supporting me and others following this journey. We were still able to support and look out for each other and not travel the road alone.

Still today, monthly get-togethers glue this group together. We also have varied activities – morning teas, lunches and barbecues – and are a cheery group that enjoys our outings and chatty times together.

We have a motto: 'In this world where you can be anything, be kind'.

I do understand the reasoning behind the cancer group's decision to a degree. Yes, while undergoing treatment, a person must practise self-care, but volunteering in that position was my self-care. Maybe having a blanket rule regarding cancer support should not be a one-size-fits-all, and it would be encouraging to see the group revisit this rule.

Do what you feel is best for you is my advice, as only you yourself can judge what is best for you.

Redefining normal

What is normal?

According to *The Oxford Dictionary*, normal is defined as 'regular, usual, typical'.

So, is this my usual state?

Of course not. Just like when I had polio, I discovered that some old stigmas still exist.

People may think someone who is living with cancer is unfit to volunteer. Some may avoid a cancer sufferer for fear of saying the wrong thing. Then there is a belief that you aren't healthy enough to continue leading a 'normal life'.

Redefining normal for me was what I felt comfortable with, not what others thought I should be doing. So many of my friends were concerned and thought I should retire from all duties in my clubs. That was certainly not the road I wanted to follow. Keeping busy was, and still is, important to me – and 'my normal'.

This intruder may have changed my life, but it cannot – I will not let it – change who I am.

As with most cancers, bladder cancer doesn't just affect the body; it impacts all aspects of your life. It is your constant companion, not one that is limited to the doctor's waiting room. I think that one of the hardest things is the unknown of its return.

How do I know it won't come back?

There is that ongoing fear of secondary cancer. My surgeon told me that bladder cancer is one type that often does recur, so there is always this anxiety for the future.

My new normal is that I have the power to shape and follow my new life's path. My new normal may mean different goals than those I had before cancer. I need to continue my journey and encourage others to do the same, using our newfound wisdom and strength.

The wisdom achieved is simple: value what you have and continue to value and enjoy life. Do not let cancer define you. Redefine yourself from what you have faced and gained strength from.

What strength have I gained? For me, remaining positive is paramount. It was important not to let this 'intruder' invade my relationships with family and friends. Birthdays and Christmases were to remain festive and full of celebration. My husband loves travelling and cycling, and it was important that he could still do these things and not think of me as a burden.

Admittedly, it was, and still is, hard at times, but this new normal is to stay my 'normal'.

My advice? Try to cross off some of the items on your bucket list and enjoy every day you can get out of bed. Greet the day with gusto.

Using humour to cope

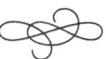

Cancer doesn't hold back, and neither should we.

I've discovered that all of the procedures involved with bladder cancer are humiliating, with no respect for your modesty.

Three months after my surgery, I was to have my first check with the surgeon. This involved a cystoscopy, a procedure whereby an instrument called a cystoscope is inserted into your bladder, allowing the surgeon to look around and check for tumour recurrence.

I'd be lying if I said I wasn't apprehensive about this visit. It would be wrong to say otherwise.

Of course I'm nervous! I'm about to be given a prediction in regards to my future health and longevity.

With all the challenges bladder cancer sufferers face, a touch of humour can shed an atom of relief. When my surgeon asked if it was okay for student doctors to be present at my cystoscopy, I agreed, despite feeling vulnerable. It really wasn't okay. The room was packed full of students viewing my nether regions. I'm not talking about one or two or three students, but around twenty or more.

I wasn't going to stop trainees from a learning situation, but I was certainly not comfortable in my head at all. So, when the surgeon returned to chat with me about the results, I blurted out how lucky he was not to have been born a woman.

He studied my face before responding sceptically, 'Oh, why is that, Jan?'.

'Well, it seems to me that, as females, at almost every stage of our lives, we have to be subjected to a situation whereby our legs are either up in the air, or we are attracting some sort of attention below,' I responded with a laugh.

'When we are born, we have our nappies changed on a regular basis. Then we become teenagers and get periods. Then we move on to sex, and some of us have babies. And now look at me!'

This wonderful man never batted an eyelid, but got down on his knees, held my hand and said, 'I'm so sorry, but we are doing everything we can to save your bladder. Your initial tumour has been completely excised, but bladder cancer is known to recur. You will be having these cystoscopies every three months for some time.'

Yes, humour can help you, in even the darkest of moments.

There were other instances where I used humour to mask my fears and embarrassment. A great example was that first infusion and the difficulty my poor nurse had with inserting the catheter. At the time, I had thought it would be a great idea if she went and got my husband and asked him for advice.

I'm sure these situations are quite usual for the doctors and nurses who deal with them every working day. I would think they understand the emotional drain on their patients, and in my experience, they do their very best to make you feel at ease.

So, never underrate the value of appropriate humour in these situations. The idea that humour and laughter are good for one's wellbeing is not new and is well debated, but I haven't found any scientific evidence to validate this.

Nevertheless, I am going to stick with the adage that laughter really is the best medicine.

Communicating with other sufferers

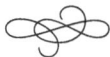

Sharing our experiences, our fears and anxieties can be really helpful. For me, I found I was not alone fighting this type of cancer.

As I began to research information about my specific cancer, it became obviously apparent that the world is focused on breast cancer and all its related support mechanisms.

This is absolutely fine, given its prevalence, but I needed to know about bladder cancer and what to expect.

Stories from bladder cancer survivors and their support mechanisms form a map, a tapestry of experiences. No one can walk this path alone, and I communicated with and spoke to many others following the same path. It proved helpful to share with others and to know I wasn't walking this road alone.

The internet is a source of information, but it isn't always reliable. Plus, bladder cancer is not just about the medical facts. It brings many emotions with it.

Chatting with other sufferers was informative, helpful and often reassuring. I needed to be aware, though, that everyone's journey was different and we don't necessarily experience the same reactions.

I did find it comforting to meet with fellow sufferers who were a long way along the road of their journey. I really wanted to find other women in similar situations, but that was difficult, as bladder cancer is not as common in women as it is in men.

Speaking with the nurse specialists, I discovered that there were five women who had recently been treated at Thames Hospital, of which two who had survived. I was one of those two.

With confidentiality paramount in the medical world, the staff could not disclose these people's names.

I did also learn that Waikato Hospital had treated eight women over the past few years, but I was unable to get any statistics as to the status of these women.

During this time, I was also privileged to meet with two wonderful men who were prepared to share their stories – something for which I am grateful for.

My husband worked with Kevin in the communications centre of the New Zealand Fire Service many years ago and they remained friends.

Kevin, now in his early seventies, had unfortunately joined the group of bladder cancer sufferers, and so we visited Kevin and his lovely wife Sandy.

With his permission, Kevin has allowed me to share details of our conversation.

Kevin's story

'We were away on holiday and had been for a really long walk. We went to a bar for a drink. I had to go to the toilet and shock – I peed blood. Within a fortnight, I had seen my doctor and then a urologist for investigation. The CT scan showed a bladder tumour, thereby bladder cancer was diagnosed.'

What were his thoughts upon diagnosis?

'Not the best. I was at retirement age and had the big decision as to whether to stay working or retire. I stayed working for a while, but with the ongoing, continual post-surgery treatment, I did retire. I told my family before the operation. They were very supportive up to and after the operation with any assistance they could do for me and back up for my wife, Sandy.'

Kevin's treatment.

'After the operation to remove the cancer, I was placed under the care of our local urologist to have three-monthly flexible cystoscopies and six-weekly BCG infusions. Having BCG treatment for so long had a worrying effect on me, as some nurses were good, others not so good, at inserting the tubes into the bladder.'

So, where is Kevin now on his cancer journey?

'Having had the cancer removed in 2016 and two years plus of BCG treatment, then three-monthly cystoscopies, then six-monthly and now twelve-monthly, I feel confident we are on top of any further complications.'

For me, this chat with Kevin was more therapeutic than fact-finding, as speaking with someone who had been along this road before me was extremely reassuring.

My sincere thanks to Kevin for his honest sharing.

∼

I also had the pleasure of meeting and speaking with a lovely couple, Bill and Judy, who I met through my garden club, and got to know even more through the Whangamatā Cancer Support Group.

Bill's story

'It was 2016, white-baiting season and high tide was to be at 3pm. I went off to my white-baiting spot and had my usual morning pee. Nothing abnormal at all. Another pee before sitting on my stool, which would be for about two hours. Still normal. Then a third, and shock as my urine had become bright red. I was so worried and packed up immediately and was off to the local medical centre. My normal doctor saw me. His demeanour was quite gruff, but he is a great doctor. Initially he said it was a urinary infection and I was started on a course of antibiotics. Nothing to worry about, I was told. My second day on antibiotics and my urine appeared clear, and so it stayed for about two weeks. Then bleeding again. More antibiotics for a further two weeks. More bleeding! And so it was off to the pathology lab, followed by a call from my doctor who asked me to come in and chat, and to expect a call from the Waikato Hospital. The subsequent cystoscopy showed a tumour and within a short time I was in hospital for surgery to remove this tumour.'

Bill underwent a transurethral resection for a bladder tumour with a follow-up of a BCG infusion. He had four-monthly checks. All was well until an unexpected return of symptoms two years later, which, thankfully, were successfully treated. Bill is now on a regime of six-monthly checks.

I asked Bill and Judy how they felt upon the diagnosis. Bill was worried; Judy was shocked. The couple told their children immediately and Judy said they were shattered, having already lost a son and brother to testicular cancer.

Now, eight years post-diagnosis, Bill and his wife are relieved to still be enjoying life. They are such a loving couple and it was heartwarming to hear their story and know they still had time to enjoy each other.

The moral I find from Bill's story is an easy one – see your doctor as soon as you notice something abnormal.

During my time in cancer support, I have met and spoken with many cancer patients from all walks of life. I have nothing but respect for the courage they all display, especially the young ones who are hoping for a longer life ahead to watch their children grow.

Cancer really does not have any boundaries. It affects anyone of any age.

So, why was it so important for me to communicate with others?

Unlike breast cancer, bladder cancer in women is one type that isn't in the public eye. I knew I needed to speak with others, so I didn't feel so alone in my battle. I was about to embark on a life-changing journey without any signposts.

My advice now to anyone in this situation is to communicate. Your oncologists, doctors and nurses are paramount in your treatment, but they are not actually sitting in your chair. This is your journey, yours alone, and, like me, only you know how you want to ride it.

Communicating and chatting with others in the same situation can be invaluable. Becoming a recluse may be chosen by some, but I feel this can be detrimental mentally. Simply chatting with others can help your positivity.

Information and knowledge are saving factors for keeping one's sanity. They can eliminate the stress that can occur from wondering about the what-ifs.

So, dance before the music is over
Live before your life is over

Reflection

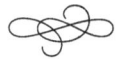

Facing any cancer, in my case bladder cancer, changes a person's way of thinking. It changes a person's view on life. You come to realise that this journey on Earth is about living every moment, celebrating milestones.

How you see the world may very well change.

Bladder cancer challenges you in ways you never ever thought you could navigate, finding strength you did not know you possessed, and realising what is important in life.

The most important lesson learned for me was acknowledging how precious family is and cherishing every moment. My biggest fear was that my grandchildren would not get to know me or even remember me.

My beautiful granddaughter, Billie, and I have a bond that will never disappear because I have been able to spend so much time with her. The twins are so young that I may not even be a memory, but their parents are so thoughtful, and with distance separating us, they make every effort to use technology and ensure we keep up with their milestones.

I have found, to my delight, that the twins bounce off each other and seem to be so advanced in many ways. I do have a strong connection with them. We treasure the times we can see them, and what a joy it is to hear them both say 'Nana' and know that they do know me.

Every step you take during your journey is a learning experience that can shape your future. Do not make it a negative experience. Instead, think of it as a pathway to enriching your life and your personal growth.

As I close these chapters of my cancer journey, I hope I will, in some small way, encourage others to share experiences and lessons learned with those beginning their journey. By doing this, you may offer a wee glimmer of light and hope for others.

Remember, and always tell yourself, that this is just a chapter in life and that life is bigger than any diagnosis you may be given.

Yes, this is simply a chapter in my life. There have been many lessons learned from both my challenges and my triumphs.

Unfortunately, this is not the end of my cancer journey as, with no permanent remission, I continue to fight this intruder in my body.

However, I am so grateful for modern medicine, the care and support I receive. Every good day is a blessing.

Take care, fellow sufferers. You are not alone. You must embrace resilience, celebrate victories and always maintain hope.

I leave my readers with this…

Life is not measured by the number of breaths we take, but by the moments that take our breath away

Bladder cancer ribbon colours.

Resources

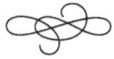

For those experiencing bladder cancer, the following organisations are useful in sourcing information from:

- National Cancer Institute
- American Cancer Society
- Malaghan Institute of Medical Research, Victoria University, Wellington, New Zealand
- Cancer Society, New Zealand.

Helpful tips

- Communicate your needs.
- Accept help when needed.
- Get professional advice if experiencing concerns, mentally or physically.
- Find a reputable acupuncturist.
- Seek helpful mechanisms such as counselling.
- Get advice from a nutritionist.
- Exercise when you can.
- Contact support groups.

Jan's support contacts in Whangamatā, New Zealand

- 🦀 Acupuncture: Katrina Wood,
  www.katrinawoodacupuncture.com
- 🦀 Havening: Penny Vaughan, Pen.jane@hotmail.com
- 🦀 Nutrition: Michelle Gilbert, MG Nutrition,
  mgnutrition@outlook.com
- 🦀 Physiotherapy: Lily Robertson, Paradise Coast Physiotherapy
- 🦀 Whangamatā Medical Centre,
  www.whangamatamedicalcentre.co.nz

About the author

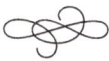

Jan Wills-Collins is an eighty-four-year-old retired nurse and health and safety consultant, spending her retirement years in the beautiful coastal town of Whangamatā, New Zealand.

In 2021, she published her memoir, *The Hidden Scars of Polio*.

Her journey with polio and its aftermath has found resonance with many people.

One would be forgiven for thinking Jan paid her dues with this illness, but this was not to be. In December 2022, Jan was diagnosed with bladder cancer.

This book is written for no other reason than to help others deal with the same situation (and possibly some self-counselling).

Other books by the author:

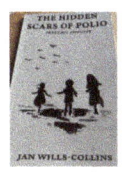 *The Hidden Scars of Polio*

References

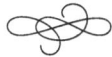

1. Cancer Council, *What is cancer?* Retrieved from https://www.cancer.org.au/cancer-information/what-is-cancer

2. Bacillus Calmette-Guerin (BCG) Treatment, Cleveland Clinic. Retrieved from https://my.clevelandclinic.org/health/treatments/17908-bacillus-calmette-guerin-bcg-treatment.

3. Secher MS, Hyldgaard J, Jensen JB. *The association between gender, stage and prognosis in bladder cancer patients undergoing radical cystectomy.* Scand J Urol. 2023 Feb-Dec;57(1-6):10-14. doi: 10.1080/21681805.2023.2166103. Epub 2023 Jan 16. PMID: 36644970.

4. Cancer Council, *What is bladder cancer?* Retrieved from https://www.cancer.org.au/cancer-information/types-of-cancer/bladder-cancer

5. Cancer Council, *Bladder cancer signs and symptoms.* Retrieved from https://www.cancer.org.au/cancer-information/types-of-cancer/bladder-cancer

6. Cancer Council, *Types of treatment.* Retrieved from https://www.cancer.org.au/cancer-information/types-of-cancer/bladder-cancer

7. Cleveland Clinic, *Bacillus Clamette-Guerin (BCG) Treatment.* Retrieved from https://my.clevelandclinic.org/health/treatments/17908-bacillus-calmette-guerin-bcg-treatment

8. Beverley Cutts, "Developing and implementing a new bladder irrigation chart," Nursing Standard, November 2, 2005. Retrieved from https://journals.rcni.com/nursing-standard/developing-and-implementing-a-new-bladder-irrigation-chart-ns2005.11.20.8.48.c3993

www.ingramcontent.com/pod-product-compliance
Lightning Source LLC
Chambersburg PA
CBHW062043290426
44109CB00026B/2719